D1712752

Everything You Need to Know About *Chemotherapy*

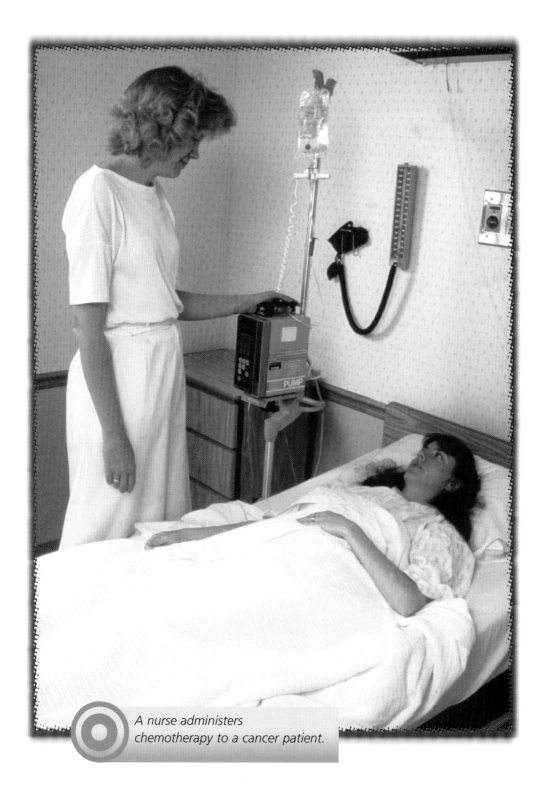

A nurse administers chemotherapy to a cancer patient.

Everything You Need to Know About *Chemotherapy*

Magdalena Alagna

The Rosen Publishing Group, Inc.
New York

Published in 2001 by The Rosen Publishing Group, Inc.
29 East 21st Street, New York, NY 10010

Library of Congress Cataloging-in-Publication Data
Alagna, Magdalena.
Everything you need to know about chemotherapy/by Magdalena Alagna. — 1st ed.
p. cm. — (Need to know library)
Includes bibliographical references and index.
ISBN 0-8239-3394-6 (lib. bdg.)
1. Cancer—Chemotherapy—Juvenile literature. 2. Tumors in children—Juvenile literature. [1. Chemotherapy. 2. Cancer—Chemotherapy.] I. Title. II. Series.
RC271.C5 A44 2001
616.99'4061—dc21

00-011392

Manufactured in the United States of America

Contents

Chapter 1   **What Is Chemotherapy?**   6

Chapter 2   **How Chemotherapy Works**   15

Chapter 3   **Side Effects**   26

Chapter 4   **What You Can Do to Help**   38

Chapter 5   **Talking with Your Doctor**   48

Glossary   55

Where to Go for Help   58

For Further Reading   61

Index   62

Chapter 1

What Is Chemotherapy?

If you are reading this book, chances are either you or someone close to you has some form of cancer and is exploring treatment options. Many patients undergoing cancer treatment receive chemotherapy. This book will explain what chemotherapy is and how it works. It will also answer questions like: How often is chemotherapy given? What can you do to lessen the side effects? How can you get the emotional support that you need? Will you be able to go on with your daily life during the time you are receiving chemotherapy? Finally, you will learn some of the questions you can ask your doctors to find out more about your treatment plan.

The Meaning of Chemotherapy

The word "chemotherapy" is made from two words: chemical and therapy. So, chemotherapy means drug treatment, or the use of drugs to treat cancer. The word "cancer" comes from "carcinos" and "carcinoma." Both of these words were coined by Hippocrates (460–370 BC), the father of medicine. In Greek, these words mean "crab." It is thought that Hippocrates chose these words because the shape of a cancerous tumor looks somewhat like a crab.

Why Chemotherapy Is Used

Basically, chemotherapy is used to stop cancer in its tracks. It is also used to relieve your symptoms and to give you a longer life by causing the disease to go into remission—the stage in which there are no active symptoms. Remission means that although the cancer may occur again, it cannot be seen on scans or X rays.

Chemotherapy works differently than surgery or radiotherapy—two other treatment options in the fight against cancer that will be explained in detail later on in this chapter. Whereas surgery and radiotherapy both work by targeting the specific area of the body where the cancer is, such as the lung or the colon, chemotherapy drugs travel throughout the whole body. This is important because it allows the drugs to reach parts of the body where the cancer cells may have spread. It is also important because using chemotherapy in combination with surgery means that fewer surgical procedures need to be done. Follow-up surgery can often be avoided if chemotherapy is used.

Combination Therapy

There are many drugs that can be used in chemotherapy. Which drug, or combination of drugs, you will be using depends on what kind of cancer you have. Most likely, you will use a combination of different drugs, not just one. This is called combination chemotherapy.

Combination chemotherapy is used because each drug that treats cancer works by treating specific symptoms and types of the disease. For example, let's say you are diagnosed with colon cancer and you take drug A, which has been proven effective in fighting this cancer. Your doctor suspects that the cancer could spread to the lining of your stomach. To limit the chances of tumors growing there, the doctor may prescribe drug B, which fights stomach cancer. Finally, you may take drug C to strengthen your body's immune system.

Combination chemotherapy also decreases the chance that you will develop a resistance to one type of drug. Developing a resistance means that the drug is no longer effective in fighting the cancer. Resistance is one reason that new drugs are being developed all the time.

Planning a Chemotherapy Treatment

Your doctor considers a few things when planning a chemotherapy treatment. Your age and general health are considered. In addition, the type of cancer you have, where it is in your body, whether it has spread, and where it has spread must also be considered. How often you get treatment and how long the treatment lasts depend on many things, including the type of cancer, the drugs used, how the cancer cells respond to the drugs, and the side effects you experience.

What Is Cancer?

In America, half of all men and one-third of all women will develop cancer during their lifetimes. In fact, millions of people today are living with cancer or have been cured of the disease.

To understand chemotherapy, it may help to know a little bit more about what cancer is and the way that it affects the body. Cancer is a disease in which abnormal cells in the body grow and multiply. There are more than 100 specific types of cancer. The one trait that all cancers share is that the cancerous cells grow and multiply at a high rate. Cancer also may involve the spread of abnormal cells.

Normal body cells grow, divide, and die in a way that maintains health and does not damage the body. When you're young, your normal cells divide faster than when you become a full-grown adult. Much of this has to do with the fact that when you reach adulthood your normal cells divide only to replace worn-out or dying cells, or to repair injuries. When you're young, normal cells divide faster because your body is growing and maturing. Cells make up all living tissue, so you need many new cells as you grow taller and stronger throughout your childhood.

But cancer cells continue to grow and divide, even though they are not serving any useful function, and can spread to other parts of the body. These cells clump together and form tumors (lumps) that may destroy normal tissue. If cells break off from a tumor, they can travel through the bloodstream or the lymphatic system to other areas of the body. When they get to a new location, they settle in and grow, eventually forming other tumors.

When a tumor spreads to a new place, it is called metastasis. Even when cancer spreads, it's still called by the name of the part of the body where it originally developed. Leukemia, however, doesn't usually form a tumor, and so in relation to other cancers, it is the exception to the rule. In leukemia, the cancer cells get into the blood and the organs that make blood—bone marrow,

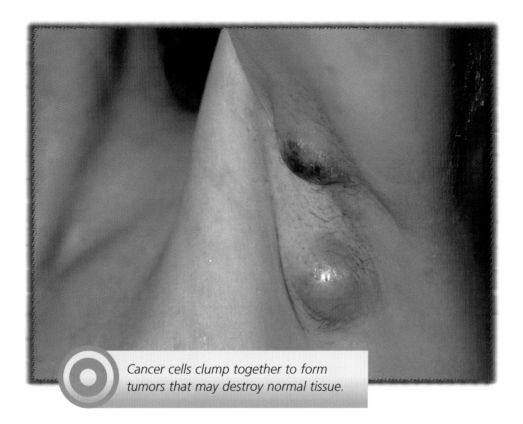

Cancer cells clump together to form tumors that may destroy normal tissue.

the lymphatic system, and the spleen. Then they circulate through other tissues, where they can build up.

It is important to remember that not all tumors are cancerous. A tumor that is cancerous is called a malignant tumor, and a tumor that is not cancerous is called a benign tumor. Benign tumors don't metastasize and are usually not life-threatening.

Chemotherapy Used with Other Treatments

Chemotherapy is extremely effective in treating cancer. It is even more effective when it is used with other

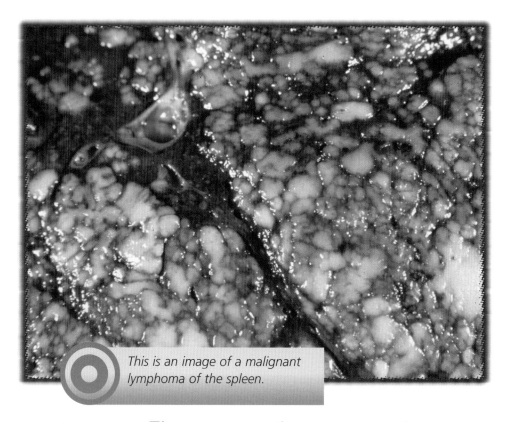

This is an image of a malignant lymphoma of the spleen.

treatments. There are two other treatments that are most often used in combination with chemotherapy to treat cancer: radiotherapy and surgery.

What Is Radiotherapy?

Radiation therapy, or radiotherapy, is the use of high-energy rays to treat disease. Radiation causes damage to cancer cells so they stop growing. With each treatment, more of the cells die and the tumor shrinks. The dead cells break down and are carried away by the blood, eventually passing out of the body. Normal cells that are exposed to radiation start to repair themselves after a few hours.

You may be concerned that radiation therapy hurts. This is not true. Radiotherapy is actually quite painless. Also, in case you are wondering, the radiation goes through your body and then passes out of your body—it does not cause you to become radioactive.

Surgery

Surgical removal of cancer is often the first and most important treatment option. The use of chemotherapy after surgery to destroy the few remaining cancer cells is called adjuvant therapy. If chemotherapy is used before surgery to shrink a tumor, it is called neoadjuvant therapy.

For a long time, the only way to treat cancer was to remove a tumor by using surgery. Even in the early part of the twentieth century, cancer could be cured only if the tumor was very small and was local. A tumor that is local stays in one place and does not spread to other areas in the body. Before chemotherapy, if the tumor was too big to be completely removed by surgery, there wasn't much that medical science could do. At that time, if tumors were too large, the invasion of surgery would be too much for the body to handle. Also, there was a danger that surgery could cause the cancer to "seed" in the incision site. When cells from a tumor break away from that tumor and attach themselves to the area where an incision was made, that is called seeding.

Today, surgery is used in combination with chemotherapy and radiotherapy. Sometimes drugs and/or radiotherapy are used to shrink tumors before surgery so that the surgery will not be so hard on the body.

In the next chapter, you will find out how chemotherapy works. This includes its effects on normal cells and on cancerous cells, and where and how chemotherapy is given.

Chapter 2

How Chemotherapy Works

There is much to know about how chemotherapy works. Do the drugs help control symptoms? Can drugs shrink tumors? Where can you get chemotherapy? In what part of the body is it given? The main thing to know is that chemotherapy drugs work on the cells in your body. Some drugs attack the cancer cells. Other drugs work to strengthen the healthy cells in your body.

The Life of a Cell

To understand how chemotherapy works, it is helpful to know some basics about the cells of the body. Everything in your body is made up of cells. A group of cells is called tissue and tissues make up all the

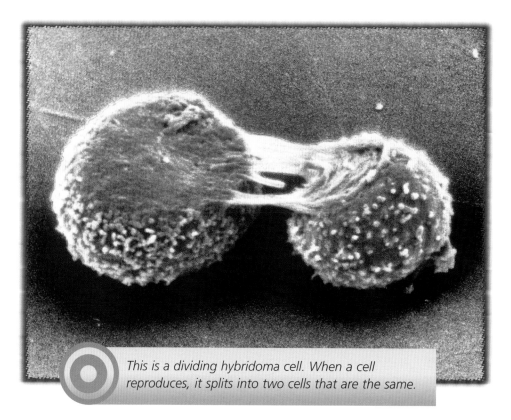

This is a dividing hybridoma cell. When a cell reproduces, it splits into two cells that are the same.

organs, the major structures of your body. Tissue stays healthy because cells grow and reproduce. New cells replace the ones that are damaged because of injury.

Both normal cells and cancerous cells go through the same cycle in order to grow and form new cells. When a cell reproduces, it splits into two cells and these two cells are exactly the same. However, cells do not divide all the time. Instead, they take time to rest in between divisions.

It is important to know about the cycle of cells because chemotherapy drugs work during specific phases of a cell's life. This means that a combination of drugs may be used to attack cancer cells so that each drug can attack the cells in a different phase. Part of developing a treatment plan is knowing when each drug should be used and which drugs are likely to work well together. Overall, this makes a complete treatment.

The Effect of Chemotherapy on Normal Cells

Chemotherapy damages cancer cells, but it also can damage normal, healthy cells. Damage to these cells is what causes the side effects of chemotherapy treatment. For instance, normal cells that divide quickly, such as blood cells and the cells of hair follicles, are more likely to be damaged by chemotherapy medications. This is why many people experience hair loss. It also is why many people experience low blood cell counts. Low blood cell counts can cause a variety of problems, such as infection. Unlike cancerous cells, however, healthy cells repair themselves quickly after being damaged by chemotherapy. In other words, in healthy cells, the damage doesn't last. Most side effects disappear once treatment is over, and many only happen on the days you actually take the drug.

The Effect of Chemotherapy on Cancerous Cells

The drugs used in chemotherapy work because they damage the material from which the cell is made. They also damage the structures that cancerous cells use to reproduce. So not only does chemotherapy attack the cancer cells that already exist, it also slows or stops the cancer cells from growing and multiplying.

A cancer treatment called biotherapy, or immunotherapy, works the way the body's natural immune system does, by attacking cancer cells. Immunotherapy drugs can work in one of two ways. Some drugs attack cancer cells so that they grow more slowly, while other drugs help your body's healthy cells become stronger so that the healthy cells can attack the cancer cells and kill them. Either way, the goal is the same: to decrease the number of cancerous cells.

Before Chemotherapy Treatment

Before your treatment, you will have blood tests, X rays, or scans. A doctor will also examine you. These tests give the doctor information about the treatment you need, and can provide a baseline picture to compare with tests done during and after the treatment, so that you will be able to see how well the treatment is working. This series of tests is also necessary to check what effects the treatment is having on your body. The doctor needs to know if there are any damaging effects on major organs such as the liver, kidneys, and heart. There also could be some damaging effects on your blood.

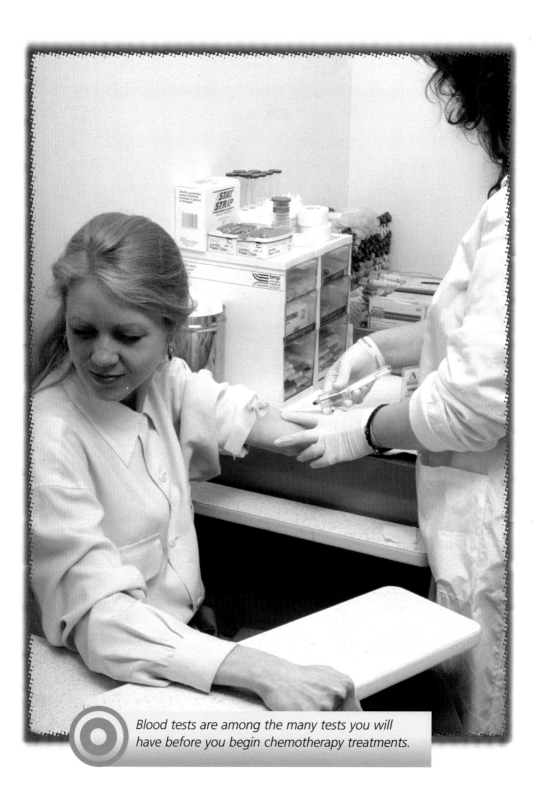

Blood tests are among the many tests you will have before you begin chemotherapy treatments.

These kinds of tests will let you know if your treatment should stay the same or if it should be changed. If it should be changed, how much should it be changed, or should it be changed completely?

The Chemotherapy Regime

Chemotherapy is usually given in several cycles. Depending on the drug or combination of drugs, each treatment lasts from a few hours to a few days, and is repeated every three or four weeks. Your doctor may refer to this as your chemotherapy regime.

As mentioned earlier, all cells, even cancer cells, rest between divisions. Chemotherapy can only attack cells that are dividing. So giving the chemotherapy as a course of treatments over a long period allows more cancer cells to be killed by the chemotherapy. The few weeks of rest between treatments also allows your body to recover from any side effects you may be experiencing.

How well your cancer responds to the chemotherapy is what will determine the number of treatments you will have. It generally takes a few months to complete your course of chemotherapy.

Where Chemotherapy Is Given

You can receive chemotherapy at a variety of places. You may get treatment as a day patient at the hospital in the outpatient department. Other chemotherapy treatments mean a short stay in the hospital, maybe overnight or for a few days. With some treatments you need to stay in the hospital for longer, perhaps for a few weeks. Other times, chemotherapy tablets can be taken at home with regular visits to the hospital out-patients department for check-ups. Where you receive chemotherapy depends on which drug or combination of drugs you are getting. It also depends on your doctor's preference and whether or not the hospital has policies about giving chemotherapy.

No matter where you get your chemo, it is very important to stick with the schedule your doctor prescribes. Otherwise, the drugs may not have their best effect. If you miss a treatment session or skip a dose of medication, call your doctor and ask for instructions about what to do next.

How Chemotherapy Is Given

Depending on the type of cancer you have and the drug or combination of drugs you are getting, your chemotherapy can be given in a number of different ways. It is your job to tell your doctor how you're feeling about the treatments. The same treatment options don't work for everyone. There are a few different ways to receive chemotherapy, so if you are uncomfortable with your method of treatment, your doctor can try another one.

Intravenously

If you are given chemotherapy intravenously, a thin needle is filled with a drug that is then injected into your vein. The vein used is usually on your hand or on your lower arm. Depending on the type of drug, or combination of drugs, intravenous, or IV, chemotherapy may be given for a few minutes, a few hours, or a few days at a time. If it only takes a few minutes, the treatment can be done in the outpatient department of the hospital. If it takes a few days, you probably will be admitted for a hospital stay. Many people who need this type of lengthy intravenous chemotherapy use pumps to take their medicine, so they can receive their treatments at home.

Another way to get intravenous chemotherapy is by using a catheter. A catheter is a thin tube that is placed into a large vein in your body. The tube stays there as long as it is needed. This type of catheter is known as a central venous catheter. Sometimes, a central venous catheter is attached to a port. A port is a small plastic or metal container placed under the skin, and surgery is required to place the port under your skin.

Orally

Chemotherapy can also be given orally, or by mouth. This type of chemotherapy can come in a pill, a capsule, or in liquid form. Basically, you swallow the drug the same way you do other medications, such as aspirin. If you're taking chemotherapy by mouth, you may take small doses every day for a few days or for many weeks or months. Then you'll have a rest period.

Pumps

Infusion pumps are now a common way of getting chemotherapy. Pumps slowly give out a designated amount of the drug over a period of time. A nurse can show you or a family member or friend how to care for the pump. Most pumps are battery operated, so you need to be careful not to get them wet. However, you will still be able to take a bath or a shower. If you have any questions about the pump, a nurse, doctor, or pharmacist can help you learn how to take care of it.

Infusion pumps work through a central line, a long plastic tube that is put into a vein in your chest. One common type of central line is called a Hickman line. The central line can stay in your vein for many months. One advantage of this is that you won't have to be stuck with needles during your chemotherapy treatment. You can also go home with a pump, so you won't have to make as many visits to the hospital.

There are some problems that could happen with your pump. For instance, you could get an infection. Keep your doctor informed of any symptoms—such as a fever—because this could signal an infection. Also, the line could get blocked. Many doctors will prescribe a drug that prevents blood clots from forming, which would result in a blocked line.

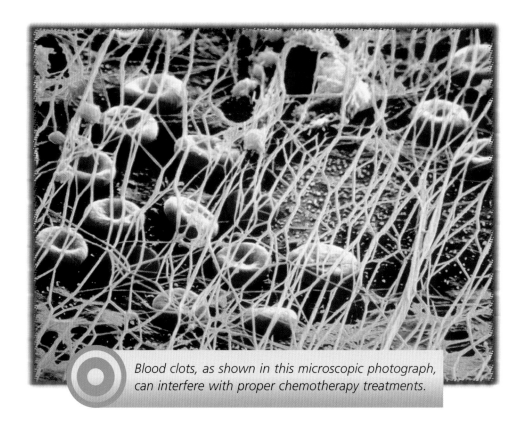

Blood clots, as shown in this microscopic photograph, can interfere with proper chemotherapy treatments.

Other Ways to Get Chemotherapy

You could get chemotherapy injected into a muscle. This is known as giving chemotherapy intramuscularly. Or you could get it injected under the skin, which is called subcutaneous chemotherapy ("sub" means under and "cutaneous" refers to skin). You might also get chemotherapy injected directly into the cancerous area. This is known as getting chemotherapy interlesionally. Finally, you can use medication topically, which means that you put the drug right on the skin.

Does Chemotherapy Hurt?

Getting chemotherapy by mouth, through the skin, or by injection usually feels the same as when you take other medications in the same ways. Starting an IV often feels like getting blood taken for a blood test. Does chemotherapy hurt? You will feel a pinprick when you are getting an injection or having an IV tube inserted, but chemotherapy shouldn't hurt. When the IV is inserted, if you have any strange sensations, such as pain, burning, coolness, or discomfort, be sure to tell the doctor or nurse.

The next chapter deals with the side effects of chemotherapy. You will find out what the short-term and long-term side effects of chemotherapy are, as well as how long they last. You will also learn what you can do to help control, lessen, and deal with the side effects of chemotherapy.

Chapter 3

Side Effects

Some people lead fairly normal lives during chemotherapy treatment. Others may feel unwell during the treatment but generally feel okay between treatments. If, for example, you are taking chemotherapy tablets at home, you may notice very little change in your everyday life. You may be able to work and carry on your usual social life. Some people even work part-time in between treatments. The bulk of this chapter describes the major side effects of chemotherapy.

Fatigue

You may feel tired during chemotherapy. That's normal. The drugs may cause it, or it also may be caused by the fact that your body is using so much energy to fight the cancer. Many times, people who are getting chemotherapy find it hard to sleep. A few nights of tossing and turning trying to get comfortable certainly can make you tired. Part of the fatigue could be caused by a mild anemia from having a lower red blood cell count than you usually do. Anemia is a condition of the blood that is caused by a low red blood cell count. Anemia can also result from having a low volume of blood, or by having low amounts of hemoglobin, the part of the red blood cell that adds pigment, or color.

If you normally have a lot of energy, feeling tired all the time can be difficult. If you feel tired from chemotherapy, there are a few things you need to remember. Keep in mind that you may not have the energy to do everything that you are used to doing. You may have to pick and choose which are the most important activities to get done in a day. It is incredibly important that you don't fight the fatigue. Take time to rest. If you have a job, see if you can work fewer hours during your treatment. Ask your family or friends to help with the chores, if possible.

If you are having trouble sleeping, your doctor may be able to give you some mild sleeping pills. Do not take any over-the-counter remedy without first asking your doctor whether it is safe to do so. Many medications limit how effectively the chemotherapy drugs can work. In fact, always check with the doctor before you take any medication, even a painkiller such as aspirin.

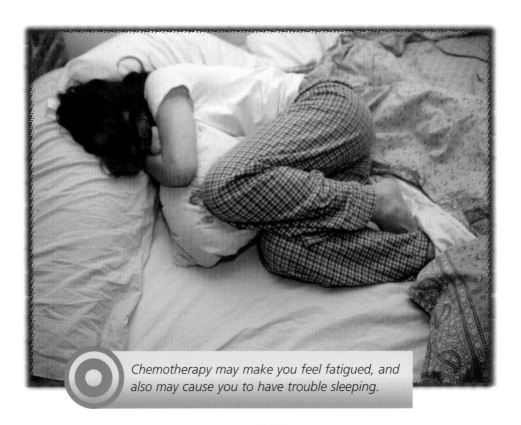

Chemotherapy may make you feel fatigued, and also may cause you to have trouble sleeping.

Chemotherapy's Effects on Bone Marrow

Bone marrow is the soft tissue found inside some bones. Bone marrow produces red blood cells (RBCs), white blood cells (WBCs), and blood platelets.

Damage to bone marrow is one of the most common side effects of chemotherapy. The number of blood cells in samples of a patient's blood will be counted regularly. This is because healthy levels of blood cells are important for many functions in the body.

Blood Cells

Knowing what the blood cells do in the body may help you to understand what it means to have a low blood cell count. WBCs help the body resist infections. Platelets help to prevent excessive bleeding by forming plugs to seal up blood vessels. RBCs bring oxygen to tissues so cells in the body can use that oxygen to turn certain nutrients into energy. When the blood cell counts are at their lowest, it means that the chemotherapy is producing severe side effects.

Low White Blood Cell Count

If the WBC count is low, be on the lookout for infections. If the WBCs are really low, patients usually are given antibiotics to reduce the risk of infection. Some of the signs of an infection are: fever, sore throat, a cough or shortness of breath, nasal congestion, shaking chills, burning during urination, and redness or swelling where an injury has taken place. If you have any of these symptoms, especially if you have a fever, contact your doctor immediately.

Low Red Blood Cell Count

Not having enough red blood cells is called anemia. People with anemia may have the following symptoms: fatigue, dizziness, headaches, irritability, shortness of breath, and increased heart rate and/or rate of breathing.

Anemia because of chemotherapy is temporary. However, blood transfusions may be needed for a while until the bone marrow is healthy enough to replace the worn-out RBCs. Because blood transfusions have some risks, doctors only do them if patients have serious symptoms of anemia.

Low Platelet Counts

People with low blood platelet counts tend to bruise easily, bleed longer than usual after minor cuts or scrapes, have bleeding gums or nose bleeds, develop either large bruises or multiple small bruises, or have serious internal bleeding (if the platelet count is very low). Low platelet counts as a result of chemotherapy are also temporary. However, they can cause serious blood loss from injury or bleeding that can damage internal organs. It is for this reason that if a patient's platelet count is very low, surgery may have to be delayed until the platelet count is more normal. The doctor won't want to risk a patient losing too much blood during surgery.

Hair Loss

Hair follicles are made of cells that grow very quickly. Therefore, they are easily affected by chemotherapy, though not everyone who gets chemotherapy will lose his or her hair. Hair loss depends on which drugs are given, how large the dose is, and how long the treatment goes on. People may experience thinning hair or complete hair loss two to three weeks after treatment begins. Loss of eyebrows, eyelashes, and other body hair is usually less than the loss of hair on the scalp.

Hair loss is almost always temporary. It is not life-threatening, but it can affect a patient's life greatly. A patient may become depressed or may experience a loss of self-confidence. The hair starts to grow again three to four months after the initial hair loss during treatment.

Appetite and Weight Loss

Loss of appetite may directly result from the effects of the chemotherapy on the body's metabolism—how the body uses calories. Decreased appetite is usually temporary. Appetite returns when treatments are over, although it may take several weeks. If you experience this side effect, talk with your doctor. There are medications that can help prevent appetite loss. Remember that proper nutrition is very important because it helps the body fight disease.

Taste Changes

Cancer treatments, and the cancer itself, can change the way you taste food. Changes in taste and smell may happen for as long as the treatment goes on. A few weeks after the treatment has ended, taste and smell should return to normal. During chemotherapy, a patient may notice either a craving for sweet food or a dislike of it. He or she may also dislike bitter tastes, or dislike tomatoes and tomato products. He or she may not like the taste of beef or pork. Some patients describe a metallic or medicinal taste in the mouth.

Nausea and Vomiting

Some chemotherapy drugs cause nausea and vomiting by irritating the stomach lining. Nausea is an unpleasant, wavelike feeling in the stomach and the back of the throat. It often comes with a feeling of weakness or dizziness, and perspiration. Symptoms of nausea and vomiting can happen immediately after treatment or within twenty-four hours after treatment, and they may continue for several days. These symptoms also can be anticipatory—anticipatory nausea happens before a treatment. Usually, it occurs because a patient remembers the nausea that he or she experienced last time as a result of chemotherapy treatment.

There are new medications to help prevent nausea and vomiting. In addition to the drugs that help with these side effects, you can try ginger in tablets or in ginger ale, relaxation exercises, or soothing music.

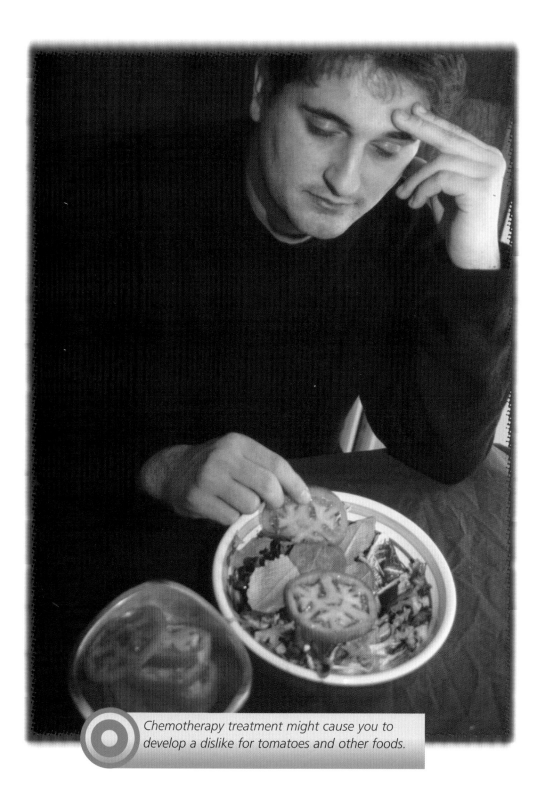

Chemotherapy treatment might cause you to develop a dislike for tomatoes and other foods.

Constipation or Diarrhea

Constipation is passing infrequent, hard, dry stool. Symptoms also may include bloating, increased gas, cramping, or pain. Although this may be a symptom of chemotherapy, factors such as depression, poor diet, not drinking enough water, and decreased physical activity can contribute to constipation, as well.

Diarrhea is passing loose or watery stools three or more times a day, with or without discomfort. Symptoms may also include gas, cramping, and bloating. Diarrhea occurs in 75 percent of chemotherapy patients. The frequency and severity will depend on which drugs are taken, how much of the drug, and for how long. Some factors, such as having a stomach tumor, being lactose intolerant (when your body can't digest dairy products), or receiving both radiation and chemotherapy, can increase the chance that you will have diarrhea.

It is always important to drink enough water, and this is especially important to remember when or if you have diarrhea. This is because the body is depleted of water more quickly and if you do not drink enough water you could become dehydrated.

Damage to the Major Organs

Although chemotherapy is efficient for fighting cancer cells, it isn't always so great for the healthy tissue in your body. Chemotherapy sometimes can affect the body's major organs. Doctors keep a careful watch on how chemotherapy drugs affect important organs.

Heart Damage

Certain chemotherapy drugs can damage the heart. Patients may feel puffy, short of breath, or dizzy. They may have an irregular heartbeat or a dry cough, or they may notice a swelling in their ankles. Those patients who smoke and those who have had radiation to the midchest area or who have existing heart problems, such as uncontrolled high blood pressure, will be at higher risk for heart damage. Doctors do tests before chemotherapy treatments to find out whether a patient has existing damage to his or her heart. Also, during treatment, heart function is checked to make sure that everything is okay and no major changes have occurred. If you have a change in heart rhythm, weight gain, or are retaining fluids, you should let your doctor know immediately.

Lung Damage

Some chemotherapy drugs cause damage to the lungs. This is more likely to happen if a patient is also receiving radiation to the chest as well as chemotherapy. Also, age seems to be a factor in this kind of tissue damage—those patients over seventy years old are at a greater risk for lung damage.

Symptoms may include shortness of breath, a dry cough, and possibly fever. If the drug that is causing the lung damage is stopped, the lung tissue can repair itself.

Liver Damage

The liver is what processes most of the chemotherapy drugs that enter the body. However, some of the drugs can cause damage to the liver. Symptoms may include a yellow coloring to the skin and the white of the eyes, fatigue, and pain under the lower part of the right ribs or right upper abdomen. Doctors must look for signs of liver damage during blood tests. Advanced age, as well as a history of hepatitis, may be risk factors for liver damage. Most often, this damage is temporary, and the liver starts to repair itself a few weeks after the chemotherapy drug is stopped.

Kidney Damage

Some drugs can affect the kidneys. Those patients who have a history of kidney problems are at greater risk for kidney damage. Symptoms may include headache, pain in the lower back, fatigue, weakness, nausea, vomiting, increased blood pressure, increased rate of breathing, change in pattern of urination, change in color of urine, an urgent need to urinate, and swelling or puffiness of the body. Blood tests should be done regularly to keep a watch on the kidneys' health.

Long-Term Side Effects of Chemotherapy

Some people can experience the side effects of chemotherapy treatment even after the treatments have stopped. These symptoms may become chronic, which means that they happen all the time, or new side effects could begin to occur. Long-term side effects depend on which drugs were taken and whether the patient received other treatment as well, such as radiotherapy.

Certain chemotherapy treatments can cause permanent damage to the body's organs. If the damage becomes obvious during the treatment, the drug will, of course, be stopped.

However, some symptoms do not appear until after the chemotherapy has been completed. Some examples of this are impaired memory, shortened attention span, seizures, hearing loss or tinnitus (ringing in the ears), or nerve damage such as numbness, tingling, or prickling sensations in the hands and feet. Also, until the immune system returns to normal, patients may be at a greater risk for pneumonia. For these reasons, and to monitor the cancer's remission, follow-up care after chemotherapy treatment is very important.

Chapter 4

What You Can Do to Help

There is a lot to know about cancer and about chemotherapy. Because of the large amount of information, many people who have cancer or whose loved ones have cancer can feel overwhelmed. They may not know exactly what they can do to help themselves or to help a loved one who is in chemotherapy treatment.

Once you sort it all out, however, there is plenty that you can do to help. You can become informed about—and practice—good nutrition. That includes knowing the pros and cons of taking vitamin supplements and herbal remedies. You can learn ways to overcome depression and anxiety, or study relaxation techniques that will help you to decrease stress. You can concentrate on talking openly and honestly about your thoughts and feelings. This will help you to maintain close relationships, to get the emotional support that you need, and to go on with your daily life.

In this chapter you will find out about all of these skills, and how you can apply them to improve either your life or the life of a loved one who is in chemotherapy treatment.

Eating Well

Practicing good nutrition is important for everyone, but it is especially important for those who are receiving chemotherapy. Eating the right kinds of foods before, during, and after treatment will help you to stay stronger and to feel better. Good nutrition will also help you to deal with the side effects of chemotherapy. It will help you to decrease your chance of infection, and to recover and heal as quickly as you can.

Eating well means eating a variety of foods from the four food groups: grains, proteins, fruits/vegetables, and dairy. The Food Guide Pyramid is a guideline to basic nutrition, and it is based on the United States Department of Agriculture (USDA) dietary guidelines. Of course, you don't have to follow the food pyramid to the letter. Instead, it is a general guide to show you how to balance your diet to include enough fruits, vegetables, fiber, and protein.

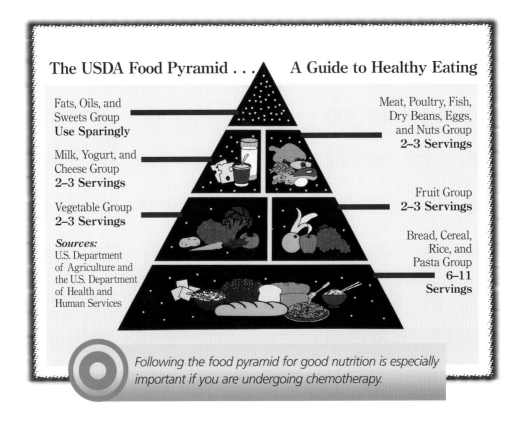

The USDA Food Pyramid . . .   **A Guide to Healthy Eating**

Fats, Oils, and
Sweets Group
Use Sparingly

Milk, Yogurt, and
Cheese Group
2–3 Servings

Vegetable Group
2–3 Servings

Sources:
U.S. Department
of Agriculture and
the U.S. Department
of Health and
Human Services

Meat, Poultry, Fish,
Dry Beans, Eggs,
and Nuts Group
2–3 Servings

Fruit Group
2–3 Servings

Bread, Cereal,
Rice, and
Pasta Group
**6–11
Servings**

Following the food pyramid for good nutrition is especially important if you are undergoing chemotherapy.

In addition, it is important to remember to drink enough water. You also may want to take vitamin supplements, especially if you are having a problem with loss of appetite. Or you may feel that you are not getting enough nutrients just from eating a normal balanced diet. However, make sure that you check with your doctor before taking any kind of vitamin, mineral, or herbal supplement. Some of these may interfere with the effectiveness of the chemotherapy or your body's natural ability to heal itself.

Healthy Eating Habits for People with Cancer

Nutrition guidelines for people with cancer are a little different than the guidelines set for healthy people, in that they focus on helping you to eat more high-calorie foods and more protein. You might be encouraged to eat or drink more milk, cheese, and cooked eggs. You also can go ahead and use all of those gravies and sauces that include butter, margarine, or oil. This will increase the calories in your style of cooking. You should also eat lots of fruit, vegetables, and whole-grain breads and cereals. Also include a moderate amount of meat, but make sure you cut back on sugar, alcohol, and salt. Some nutritionists suggest that for those patients having a problem with diarrhea, high-fiber foods are best eaten in moderation.

Following these special nutrition guidelines will help you to build up strength. Then it will be easier to withstand the effects of the cancer and its treatment. When you are healthy, you probably don't think much about getting the nutrients that you need. You may easily get enough nutrients by following your normal balanced diet. However, when you are in chemotherapy, getting nutrients may be challenging. There may be side effects from the treatment that interfere with your appetite. If you don't feel well, you may not feel like eating.

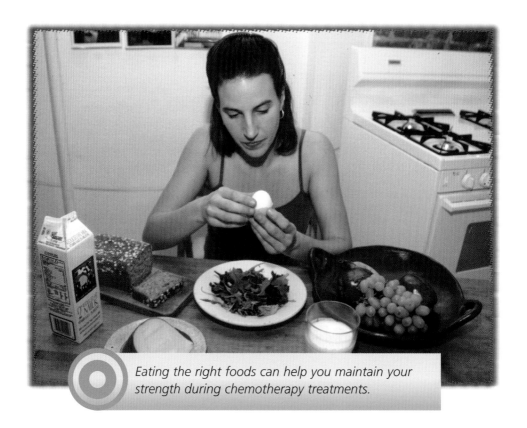

Eating the right foods can help you maintain your strength during chemotherapy treatments.

More Helpful Hints on Eating Healthy During Chemotherapy

Hint #1   On the days that you have chemotherapy treatment, it is good to have a light snack before treatment. Many people find that this keeps up their strength.

Hint #2 Also, many chemotherapy treatments are given in the outpatient department of the hospital. These treatments could take minutes, or they could take several hours. Plan ahead and bring a light meal or some snacks with you.

Hint #3 If side effects make eating meals difficult, try eating many small snacks during the day. On the days that you are feeling particularly well, make the most of it and try to eat bigger meals.

Hint #4   Foods that are high in fat, greasy, or fried are not as easy to digest, so you may find that they upset your stomach. You might want to keep foods of this type to a minimum.

Herbs, Vitamins, Minerals, Antioxidants, and Supplements

Many people want to participate more actively in their treatment. One of the ways in which they choose to do this is by taking herbs, vitamins, or mineral supplements. These have been described as alternative therapies. However, you should know that there is no medical evidence that these methods are effective.

Herbal medicine—the use of herbs to prevent or treat disease—has been practiced for thousands of years. Herbs are technically defined as the leaves of a plant, while the rest of the plant is called a botanical. Herbs and botanicals are available in many forms. These include pills, liquid extracts, and teas. Many of these products are safe to use. However, there are some that may interfere with the effectiveness of chemotherapy. Do not take any herbal product without checking with your doctor first.

Vitamin and mineral supplements can help give you the recommended amount of nutrients. This is especially true if you experience a loss of appetite as a side effect of chemotherapy. A supplement that contains 100 percent of the recommended daily allowance of most nutrients—a multivitamin, for instance—can be a safe bet.

Some cancer patients take large amounts of vitamins, minerals, and supplements. They think that this will help their immune systems fight their diseases. In fact, some of these products can do more harm than good. They can reduce the effectiveness of the chemotherapy treatment. Again, always check with your doctor before taking any of these products.

Nutrition After the Treatment Ends

When chemotherapy treatments are finished, you may need to adjust your diet once again. Remember that you may have needed extra protein, calories, and fat in your diet to help you keep strong during chemotherapy. Now that the treatment is finished, you may want to go back to eating balanced amounts of protein, carbohydrates, fruits, and vegetables. You probably will want to reduce your fat intake to a level that is within the suggested daily allowance on the USDA Food Guide Pyramid.

Here are some suggestions to help you stick to a healthy diet:

◎ Choose a variety of foods from the four food groups.

◎ Try to eat at least five servings of fruit and vegetables a day.

◎ When choosing carbohydrates, choose whole-grain, high-fiber ones such as brown rice instead of white rice, whole-wheat bread instead of white bread.

◎ Try baking or broiling food more often than frying.

◎ Try some beans or some soy products instead of having meat.

◎ Choose low-fat dairy products.

What You Can Do to Help a Loved One Undergoing Chemotherapy

Perhaps a loved one of yours has cancer and is in chemotherapy treatment, and you want to know what you can do to help him or her. You can start by offering to help around the house or by running small errands. People who are undergoing chemotherapy may be tired from the treatment. They probably will not be up to their usual strength. Even if you can't drive yet, you can still help around the house. A loved one will appreciate it if some small chores, such as feeding pets or taking clothing to the dry cleaner, can be taken care of by someone else.

You can also offer to talk about the treatment. Many times, people who are undergoing chemotherapy will want to talk about their treatment. They may feel shy about doing so because they may worry that loved ones will not want to talk about it. While they talk to you, try to listen with an open mind and an open heart.

Talking openly about cancer and about chemotherapy will help a loved one feel that you support him or her emotionally. Remember that it is also okay if a loved one does not want to talk about treatment.

One of the most important things you can do is try to keep your relationship as close to normal as you can. People undergoing chemotherapy don't want loved ones to treat them like invalids. Try to keep your loved one's spirits bright by doing fun things with him or her. Just remember that his or her strength may not be what it usually is—you may have to play a board game rather than a basketball game.

Coping with Your Own Feelings When a Loved One Has Cancer

When a loved one has cancer, you may experience many feelings all at once. This is completely natural. You may start to worry that you are at risk for cancer,

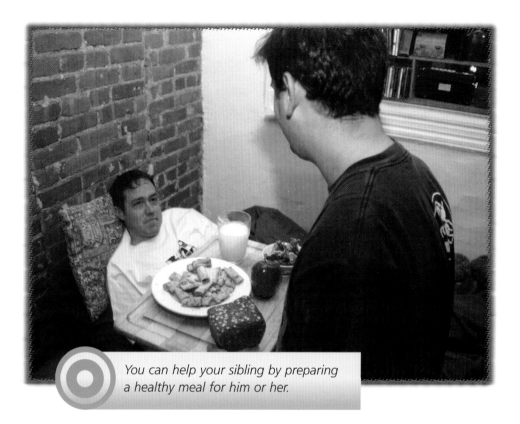

You can help your sibling by preparing a healthy meal for him or her.

not in the sense that cancer is "catching," or contagious, but in the sense that bad things can happen to good people. You may feel guilty for feeling well when someone you love is sick, or you may not want to take time to do your own thing because you think most of your time should be spent with your loved one.

It is important, however, not to neglect your own needs. Listen to your feelings, and then talk out those feelings with supportive friends or family members. It is important for you to take time for yourself and for you to continue to enjoy your life. Not only is this good for you, but it will make you more cheerful and patient when dealing with a loved one who has cancer.

Chapter

5

Talking with Your Doctor

Cancer is a disease that can make you feel depressed and powerless. But many people believe that the treatment is worse than the disease! This is not true. A tumor that is left untreated can grow until it limits the functions of one of your major organs. Cancer is much harder to treat at this later stage, but even with advanced forms of cancer, treatment can be given to manage the symptoms, such as bone pain. Treatment always should be your first plan of attack.

Open Communication

One of the ways in which you can overcome the feeling of powerlessness is to talk openly with your doctor. This is one of the most important ways you can participate in your treatment. It is especially important to keep the lines of communication open with your doctor because he or she needs to know how you feel at all times in order to prepare an effective treatment plan.

Chemotherapy drugs have a narrow range of how they can be taken, meaning they need to be prescribed specifically for you. The drugs usually are prescribed based on either your body weight or on your height and weight. If you take too low a dose, the treatment may not be effective. But if you take too large a dose, the side effects will be worse and can even be life-threatening. It is important to remember that you must always tell your doctor about any side effects that you experience.

Getting the Facts

To be able to communicate effectively, it is important to find out certain things about chemotherapy. You can find out about the tests you may need. You can help the doctor structure your treatment plan. Learning what goes into making decisions about a treatment plan will help you to follow your plan precisely and faithfully.

A Brief on Alternative Therapies

A little research will show you that there are many alternative remedies available for cancer treatment. However, not all of these remedies have been proven effective. Everything from vitamin C to shark cartilage to guided imagery has been promoted as a cure for cancer. It can be difficult to tell what is truly helpful and what is not—always check with your doctor.

General Treatment Plans

Most often, chemotherapy is given in cycles. A cycle may involve one dose, and then several days or weeks without treatment. The time without treatment enables the normal tissues in the body to recover from the effect of the drug(s). If more than one drug is used, the treatment plan will specify which drug is given at what time and in how many cycles. The treatment plan coordinates all the cycles of the different drugs given. The number of cycles can be determined before the treatment starts, because the cycles may be determined by the kind of cancer you have. However, cycles may be changed during the treatment. The side effects from your treatment may be different from those your doctor expected. This is one more reason why it is so important to talk to your doctor about the way the treatment is affecting you.

What Is a Clinical Trial?

If you want to try a new treatment for cancer, you may want to participate in a clinical trial. Clinical trials test new treatments, and might include surgery, radiation therapy, or chemotherapy. A clinical trial is an experiment. Sometimes a clinical trial involves a group of people who all receive the same experimental treatment so that doctors can find out the effects of the treatment on tumors and how patients react to the treatment.

If you want to sign up for a clinical trial, you should know a few things. One is that you may not be given the experimental drug. However, you will not know that one way or the other during the clinical trial. Patients in a clinical trial don't know whether they are receiving the established drug or the experimental drug. Also, the experimental treatment may not be the most effective treatment. It is important to remember that the medically accepted treatment for your type of cancer is the best scientifically tested treatment available.

If you talk to your doctor, you can also learn how effective chemotherapy is for the kind of cancer that you have. You can learn about the various drugs that are used in chemotherapy. You can find out whether there is an alternative treatment option for your type of cancer. Asking questions will help you know what to expect. This will greatly reduce the fear, stress, and anxiety about your treatment. Asking questions also helps you to focus your mind. That can help reduce the risk of becoming depressed.

Here are questions that you can ask your doctor:

◎ **What is the goal of chemotherapy for my cancer? What kinds of tests will I need?**

◎ **How often will I have tests once my treatment starts?**

◎ **How long does it usually take to see the results of treatments?**

◎ **How will you inform me of the results?**

◎ **What is your plan for my treatment?**

◎ **Will I take just one drug or a combination of drugs?**

◎ **Will I have surgery as well as chemotherapy?**

◎ **Will I have radiation therapy in addition to chemotherapy?**

◎ What are the chances that the chemo-therapy will work?

◎ Are there other treatments that will work as well as chemotherapy?

◎ How will I know if the chemotherapy is working?

◎ How do the side effects of chemotherapy compare with those of other treatments?

◎ How will I receive chemotherapy?

◎ How can I prepare for the treatment to decrease my chances of side effects?

◎ What changes will I have to make in my daily activities, including what I eat?

◎ What support services are available in my area?

You may have to take notes during your talks with the doctor. Don't feel shy about asking questions and writing down the answers. There will be a lot of important information being conveyed, and you will want to remember it all. You also may want to take a relative or friend with you to your doctor's appoint-ments. A loved one can remind you of the questions you want to ask. The American Cancer Society may also be able to answer many of your questions, so please check out the contact information listed in the Where to Go for Help section of this book.

Knowing what chemotherapy is and how it works, as well as how to deal with its side effects, gives you not only knowledge, but a sense of control over your life. This is important because cancer is a disease that often makes those who suffer from it feel afraid and powerless. Many people think that there isn't anything that they can do. They may think that whatever they do will not help much. But now you know how wrong that is. There is so much you can do, and as this book has explained, taking care of your health and learning all you can about your treatment are two of the most important steps you can take.

Glossary

adjuvant therapy Anticancer drugs or hormones given after surgery and/or radiation to help prevent the cancer from coming back.

anemia Having too few red blood cells. Symptoms of anemia include feeling tired, weak, and short of breath.

benign A term used to describe a tumor that is not cancerous.

biological therapy Treatment to stimulate or restore the ability of the immune system to fight infection and disease. Also called immunotherapy.

blood count The number of red blood cells, white blood cells, and platelets in a sample of blood; also called a complete blood count.

bone marrow   The inner, spongy tissue of bones, where blood cells are made.

cancer   A general term for more than 100 diseases in which abnormal cells grow out of control.

catheter   A thin, flexible tube through which fluids enter or leave the body.

central venous catheter   A special thin, flexible tube placed in a large vein. It remains there for as long as it is needed to deliver and withdraw fluids.

chemotherapy   Drugs used to treat cancer.

clinical trials   Medical research studies conducted with volunteers.

combination chemotherapy   The use of more than one drug to treat cancer.

infusion   Slow intravenous delivery of a drug or a fluid.

intralesional   Directly into the cancerous area.

intramuscular   Into a muscle.

intravenous   Into a vein.

leukemia   A type of cancer in which there is an abnormal amount of white blood cells in the tissues and/or in the blood.

malignant   A word used to describe a cancerous tumor.

metastasis   When cancer cells break away from their original site and spread to other parts of the body.

neoadjuvant therapy Chemotherapy that is used before surgery to shrink a tumor.

platelets Special blood cells that help to stop bleeding.

radiation therapy Cancer treatment with radiation (high-energy rays).

red blood cells Cells that supply oxygen to tissues throughout the body.

remission The partial or complete disappearance of the signs and symptoms of a disease.

subcutaneous Under the skin.

tissue A group of cells.

tumor An abnormal growth of cells or tissues.

white blood cells The blood cells that fight infection.

Where to Go for Help

American Cancer Society
1599 Clifton Road NE
Atlanta, GA 30329-4251
(800) ACS-2345 (227-2345)
Web site: http://www.cancer.org

American Dietetic Association
216 West Jackson Boulevard
Chicago, IL 60606-6995
(312) 899-0040
Web site: http://www.eatright.org

National Cancer Institute
NCI Public Inquiries Office
Building, 31, Room 10A13
31 Center Drive, MSC 2580

Bethesda, MD 20892-2580
(301) 435-3848
Web site: http://www.nci.nih.gov

National Coalition for Cancer Survivorship
1010 Wayne Avenue, Suite 770
Silver Spring, MD 20910-5600
(877) NCCS-YES (622-7937)
Web site: http://www.cansearch.org
e-mail: info@cansearch.org

In Canada

Canadian Cancer Society
10 Alcorn Avenue, Suite 200
Toronto, ON M4V 3B1
(416) 961-7223
(888) 939-3333
Web site: http://www.cancer.ca

Childhood Cancer Foundation Canada—Candlelighters
Suite 401, 55 Eglinton Avenue East
Toronto, ON M4P 1G8
(416) 489-6440
(800) 363-1062
Web site: http://www.candlelighters.ca
e-mail: staff@candlelighters.ca

National Cancer Institute of Canada
10 Alcorn Avenue, Suite 200
Toronto, ON M4V 3B1
(416) 961-7223
Web site: http://www.ncic.cancer.ca
e-mail: ncic@cancer.ca

WEB SITES

Association of Cancer Online Resources (ACOR)
http://www.acor.org

Canadian Cancer Research Group
http://www.ccrg.com

Cancer News on the Net
http://www.cancernews.com

Cancer Organizations in Canada
http://www.healthcastle.com/org_canada.shtml

CancerResources
http://www.cancerresources.com

For Further Reading

Capossela, Cappy, and Sheila Warnock. *Share the Care: How to Organize a Group to Care for Someone Who Is Seriously Ill.* New York: Simon and Schuster, 1995.

Dollinger, Malin, Ernest H. Rosenbaum, and Greg Cable. *Everyone's Guide to Cancer Therapy*, 3rd ed. Kansas City, MO: Andrews McMeel Publishing, 1998.

McKay, Judith, and Nancee Hirano. *The Chemotherapy and Radiation Therapy Survival Guide.* Oakland, CA: New Harbinger Publications, 1998.

Morra, Marion, and Eve Potts. *Choices*, 3rd ed. New York: Avon Books, 1994.

Yount, Lisa. *Cancer.* San Diego: Lucent Books, 1999.

Index

A
adjuvant therapy, 13
American Cancer Society, 53
anemia, 27, 29–30

B
biotherapy, 18
blood/bloodstream, 10, 12, 17, 18,
    25, 27, 28, 29, 30
blood cells, 27, 28, 29–30
    low counts, 17, 27, 29
blood test, 18, 25, 36
bone marrow, 10, 28, 30

C
cancer
    alternative therapies for, 43, 50
    different types of, 7, 8, 9, 21, 52
    spread of, 8, 9, 10–11, 13
    statistics on, 9
    what it is, 9–11
catheter, 22

cells
    basics of, 15–16
    division of, 9–10, 16, 17, 18, 20
chemotherapy
    after receiving, 37, 39, 44
    before receiving, 18–20, 35, 39
    combination therapy, 8, 17, 20, 21
    definition of, 7
    effect on cancerous cells, 17–18
    effect on normal cells, 17
    helping yourself during,
        38–45, 54
    how it's given, 21–24
    when loved one undergoes, 38,
        45–47
    with other treatments, 11–14, 34,
        35, 37
    pain involved, 25
    plan/treatment, 9, 17, 18, 20, 49, 50
    purpose of, 7–8
    regime/how often given, 17, 20,
        21, 22, 23, 50

side effects, 17–18, 20, 26–37, 39, 41, 43, 44, 49, 50
  talking about, 38–39, 46, 48–49
  where it's given, 20–21, 22, 42
clinical trials, 51

D
depression, overcoming, 38, 48, 52
diarrhea, 34, 41
dizziness, 29, 32, 35
doctor, 9, 18, 21, 23, 25, 29, 30, 35, 51
  asking questions of your, 6, 21, 27, 31, 35, 40, 44, 48–49, 50, 52–53

F
fatigue, 26–27, 29, 36, 45

H
hair loss, 17, 30–31
heart, 18, 29, 35

I
immune system, 8, 18, 37, 44
infection, 17, 23, 29, 39
injections, 24, 25
IV (intravenous), 22, 25

K
kidneys, 18, 36

L
leukemia, 10
liver, 18, 36
loss of appetite/weight loss, 31, 40, 41, 44
lung, 7, 35–36
lymphatic system, 10

M
metastasis, 10, 11

N
nausea, 32, 36
neoadjuvant therapy, 13
nutrition, getting proper, 31, 34, 38, 39–43, 44–45

O
organ damage, 18, 34–36, 37

P
pumps, 22, 23

R
radiotherapy, 7, 12–13, 14, 34, 35, 37, 51
remission, 7, 37

S
scans, 7, 18
seeding, 13
stomach, 8, 32, 34, 43
surgery, 7, 8, 12, 13–14, 30, 51

T
taste changes, 31–32
tissue, 10, 11, 15–16, 28, 29, 34, 35, 36
tumors, 8, 10, 11, 12, 13, 14, 15, 34, 48, 51

V
vitamins/herbal supplements, 38, 40, 43–44
vomiting, 32, 36

X
X rays, 7, 18

About the Author

Magdalena Alagna is a writer and editor living in New York City.

Photo Credits

Cover © Custom Medical Stock Photo, Inc.; p. 2 © SIU/Peter Arnold, Inc.; p. 11 © LI, Inc./Custom Medical Stock Photo, Inc.; p. 12 © Dr. F. C. Skvara/Peter Arnold, Inc.; p. 16 © David Scharg/Peter Arnold, Inc.; p. 19 © Amethyst/Custom Medical Stock Photo, Inc.; p. 24 © Volker Steoer/Peter Arnold, Inc.; pp. 28, 33, 42, 47 by Kristen Artz; p. 40 © Leonard Lessin/Peter Arnold, Inc.

Design and Layout

Thomas Forget

616.99   Alagna, Magdalena
ALA   Chemotherapy

6/03	**DATE DUE**		